BROKEN BODIES

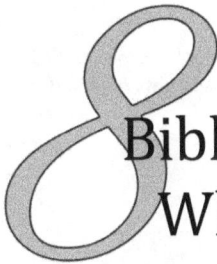

8 Biblical Reasons for Why We Get Sick

Davis McGuirt, MDiv, DVM
Heather Geisel

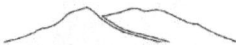

Blue Ridge Books, LLC

Blue Ridge Books, LLC
PO Box 4623 Lynchburg, VA

McGuirt, Davis.
Broken Bodies: 8 Biblical Reasons for Why We Get Sick / by Davis McGuirt and Heather Geisel

ISBN 978-0-9987481-1-5

About the cover

Jesus holding Jarius' daughter (Mark 5:21-43).

Contact Information

The author can be reached at *dmcguirt@liberty.edu.*

Contents

When the sun was setting, all those who had any that were sick with various diseases brought them to Him; and He laid His hands on every one of them and healed them.

Luke 4:40

Introduction

...Joseph was told, "Indeed your father is sick."

Genesis 48:1

I turned out of the hospital parking garage and merged into the city traffic. I had some difficulty seeing through the tears welling up in my eyes. The warm night air felt good against my arm and face, urging me to forget that moments earlier I had stood in the hospital's surgical ward. I had been listening but barely comprehending the two doctors as they explained that my Dad had inoperable cancer.

It was supposed to be a simple procedure. He had undergone surgery to remove a kidney, which – they thought – was the cause of his vomiting. When they saw the cancer and how extensive it was they stopped the surgery and just closed him up.

It fell on me to tell Dad about it when he awoke from the anesthesia. Learning that my dad had terminal cancer took me and my family completely by surprise, and now all I could manage was a heart-felt cry toward heaven. "Help," I said. "Help us, Jesus."

The next weeks and months took me along a journey of exploration in search of an explanation. I was hungry for answers, even as my dad got sicker and was put on an unwilling fast. Shortly after graduating seminary, in 1996, I had jotted down reasons I had seen from the Word of God about why people get sick. Over the next several years I thought about those reasons as I pastored a church and served the Lord in various churches, but when my dad got sick, things I had pondered theoretically for years suddenly took on new meaning. I needed to make sense of his illness, and his sickness did help clarify my thoughts on human disease and suffering. In 2014, the Lord provided help for me (in Heather Geisel) to put those thoughts on paper. You are holding the result in your hands.

I believe that our Lord wants us to understand as much as possible about disease, sickness, and dying. With that understanding our trust and faith in Him will grow. What follows are several biblical explanations for why people get sick.

BROKEN BODIES

1

SICK BECAUSE OF SIN'S ENTRANCE

Wherefore, as by one man sin entered into the world, and death by sin; and so death passed upon all men, for that all have sinned.

Romans 5:12

The first couple to get sick on the earth, Adam and Eve, had been placed in a perfect sin-free Garden. They had been warned not to eat of a certain tree of the knowledge of good and evil because "the day you eat of it you shall surely die (Genesis 2:17)." This was a real tree with real fruit, but one that had extreme spiritual significance. They were deceived by the serpent, and we are affected by it to this day. Adam and Eve didn't die immediately, but things were set in motion that day that were unstoppable. Physical death entered the world that day. Spiritual death also entered creation that day (Romans 5:12). The Hebrew word for sin means *missing the mark*. Adam and Eve missed the mark of what God had for them, and so have we. This is what is called by theologians the Fall of Man.

Sin's entrance into the world must have been a catastrophic event, marring such a beautiful perfect creation. The sin-affected world is all we have ever seen, and that makes it difficult to imagine how things looked before the Fall of Man. The natural world retains some of the original beauty. There are places on the earth that are especially blessed, and people recognize this. Pretty trees, mountains, and gardens lift our spirits. Is it God's grace that these places show hints of the Garden of Eden? Even these sights are touched by Sin. Sin has affected every part of the natural world and the ones who inhabit it. As a result, our bodies break down, decay, get sick, fail, wear out, and finally quit, just as they did for Adam and Eve.

Solomon, David's son, asked God to give him wisdom (literally a *hearing heart*) when he became king of Israel (1 Kings 3:9). He saw God in a dream at Gibeon, and it pleased God to give him wisdom unlike anyone before or after him. Infused with divine wisdom Solomon made many wise observations about death and the shortness of life. He wrote the book in the Bible called Ecclesiastes. In that book he said, "No one has power over the spirit to retain the spirit, and no one has power in the day of death. There is no discharge in that war." (Ecclesiastes 8:8). As Solomon's father, King David, neared death he used this phrase: "I go the way of all the earth…" (1 Kings 2:2). Many people are uncomfortable talking about death, but what these wise men wrote in the Bible should motivate us to search for and secure spiritual wisdom to face the afterlife.

There was no one else like Moses who knew God face to face. He was chosen to deliver Israel out of Egypt. He was the one person through whom God revealed the Ten Commandments. Even though he had a few missteps he was highly honored by God. He faced challenges leading God's people out of Egypt and through the wilderness. At times his congregation rebelled and resisted his leadership. During one of these rebellions he used a phrase "the common fate of all men." We must be prepared for what Moses called the common fate of all men! As soon as we are born we begin what Moses called, in the only Psalm attributed to him, our "numbered days." (Psalm 90).

With the Fall of man and Sin's devastating entrance into the world, disease and death spread through creation. Many people are unaware of this biblical explanation given to us and are puzzled over why people get sick. When Solomon prayed at the dedication of the temple he said every man "knows the plague of his own heart" (1 Kings 8:38). Sin is like an illness that has infected the world and every person in it! Sin brought all types of illnesses with it into this world and made everyone susceptible to sickness.

This spiritual reality shows up in the natural world as the certainty of death, and it is manifested through certain disease agents: viruses, bacteria, parasites, fungi, cancers, trauma, autoimmune conditions, etc. Man has done great work over the last century to understand the biological causes of sickness, but it is the theological ones that need investigating! Understanding biological causes may bring temporary comfort, but understanding spiritual ones can bring lasting wisdom.

Sin's entrance into the world has changed and has influenced or touched man's lifespan. We know that God set man's age limit at 120 years in Genesis 6:3. We observe that most people will die a natural death from some cause. The exceptions are Elijah, Enoch, and the saints who will be taken directly to heaven in the last days. This inevitable natural death is acknowledged in the Word of God and provides the motivation for us to be ready.

Solomon said that one event happened to all, whether they were wise or foolish (Ecclesiastes 2:14). He saw man's fate to be common with the beasts, too, and that's humbling! "Time and chance happen to all." (Ecclesiastes 9:11).

People get sick and die, no matter how spiritual they are! The man who was healed by Peter and John at the Beautiful Gate was lame "from his mother's womb" (Acts 3:2). He was not committing sins in the womb, although he could be understood as having a sinful nature. His illness was the result of Sin affecting all of creation.

Even great people of the Bible fell sick. Isaac declared that he was old and did not know the day of his death (meaning the day was at hand), even though he was the great patriarch through which all the nations would be blessed (Genesis 27:2). Asa, who was overall a great king, became diseased in his feet toward the end of his life (1 Kings 15:23). No matter how great we are before God, we may fall ill, as Elisha did in 2 Kings 13:14. This is the same Elisha that raised people from the dead! David describes a generous promise for a generous man in Psalm 41. He says the Lord will strengthen this person

8

on his sickbed who has been so considerate to the poor. Generous, godly people still get sick.

When we see sick people there is something in us that longs for an explanation, longs for an answer, longs for comfort or closure. One of the earliest mentions of illness leading to death is when Jacob declared that his children and young animals could die from over-exertion if pushed too hard traveling. (Genesis 33:13). Our bodies have limitations in this created world. There are people who are sick or injured because they pushed themselves too hard, like Jacob's flocks. There is no deep, mysterious reason why they are afflicted, they have simply gone beyond their physical limitations. Those who don't acknowledge God struggle with sickness and death, but as we just saw, godly people can get sick, too. Like it or not, the presence of illness all around us is evidence that the Bible is true and that we all need the healing ministry of our Lord and, ultimately, salvation. This is why we have the gospel! The certainty of death, and its harbinger, illness, should be a very strong motivation for understanding spiritual things and the afterlife.

There is hope. Jesus gave Himself to overcome Sin and its accompanying death. Paul said it this way: the creature itself would be delivered from the bondage of corruption one day. He said creation (of which man is a part) was, in fact, "groaning and travailing in pain" for the day of release (Romans 8:22). What a great day that will be!

All the other categories of illness fall under this first one, Sin's Entrance. Specific Sins (Chapter2) emanate from our sin nature which results from the Fall. The Devil and his demons accompanied the entrance of Sin into our world and have affected people since (Chapter 3). Church discipline exists because man goes astray due to sin (Chapter 4). Sometimes a person's illness causes them, or a loved one, to become interested in the kingdom of God (Chapter 5). The Word was given to help us combat sin, but it also contains curses and prophecies that involve sickness (Chapter 6). The nation of Israel was given special blessings along with much responsibility, but when she went astray (due to sin) she was often rebuked through illness (Chapter 7). Sadly, individuals may get sick simply from being caught up in national rebellion, or due to persecution, the sinful behavior of others. Finally, people may get sick to bring glory to God (Chapter 8), sometimes through healing which shines a bright light in sin's darkness. God sometimes validates his sin-fighters – the prophets and ministers – by allowing them to heal others from sickness.

Illness has a way of invading or intruding into our lives, causing us to think about the afterlife. It is God's grace that we can appreciate mortality. He has "set eternity in our hearts." (Ecclesiastes 3:11). We must think about death, even we who "cannot keep ourselves alive." (Psalm 22:29) This healthy fear of death can drive us to our Savior. When we find Him we can share the cry of Lazarus' sisters: "Lord, behold, the one whom you love is sick!"

2

SICK BECAUSE OF SPECIFIC SINS

When I kept silent, my bones grew old through my
groaning all the day long. For day and night
Your hand was heavy upon me.

Psalm 32:3

Jackie was a young, good-looking, athletic man who had many opportunities to date girls in college in the 1980s. Unfortunately, he had many (unmarried) sexual relationships during that time and somewhere picked up a sexually transmitted disease. The virus took an unusual clinical manifestation, invading his spinal cord and causing severe pain every few months. The pain has plagued him since college. It has almost driven him to suicide, and caused his early retirement (in his forties) and disability. The last time I spoke with him he showed no interest in God and seemed resentful of his situation.

We saw in the last chapter how disease and death are related to Sin. That is, we have real disease-causing agents unleashed due to Sin entering our world in the Garden of Eden.

Sin's Entrance in the Garden can be thought of as a result of a specific sin: *the day you eat of the fruit you will die!* Sadly, this direct warning stopped neither Adam nor us from sinning. The relationship of disease and death to specific sins is more complex. God has revealed to man in His Word what sin is (remember, *missing the mark*). We would not know what sin is except for what is revealed or defined as such in the Bible (the Word of God is the "mark"). The commands of the Bible are given to show us specifically what sin is. For unbelievers the revelation of their sins should result in their conviction and turning to Jesus Christ, the Redeemer. For the believer, re-vealed sins are there to guide us and keep us faithful. God sometimes chastens and rebukes believers to encourage us, correct us, stop us, or aid our rededication. In His sovereignty He uses punishment to get us to realize sin is real and has con-sequences. For either believer or unbeliever, if our specific sins have brought condemnation then they should ultimately lead us to our Savior. Not all sin is immediately punished, and that can be confusing to both believers and unbelievers.

We are all guilty before God and need a Savior, and it's not as if we need a disease to show us that (although some people seem to require this to get their attention)! *There are diseases, however, that are directly related to sinful activities.* Specific sins do sometimes carry real medical consequences. Specific sins can cause us to become ill. There are passages in the Bible that show this cause and effect.

Some of the individual sins that incur direct penalties are sexual. The earliest mention of this in the Bible may be Abimelech's house, healed through prayer from closed wombs (Genesis 20:17). That seemed to be a warning against

12

adultery. When an unbeliever commits specific sexual sins he may receive a penalty. If an immoral man interacts with an immoral woman he can get sexually transmitted diseases. That can, the Word says, "cause a man to mourn when his flesh and body are consumed" (Proverbs 5:11). Paul acknowledged in the New Testament that homosexuals receive a penalty in themselves when they engage in that behavior (Romans 1:27). People who are involved in criminal sexual activity sometimes get sick or injured as part of the life they've chosen or been forced into. The man who was having a sexual relationship with his father's wife was to be turned over to Satan "for the destruction of the flesh (1 Corinthians 5:1)." Jesus Himself gave advice in the book of Revelation to several churches. The Church at Thyatira was warned about Jezebel (a very wicked woman) and her sexual immorality and that she would be "cast onto a sickbed." Some of our churches contain people committing similar sexual immorality.

David's son's death after a short illness is a very sad but instructive event recorded in the Bible showing the result of the specific sin of adultery (2 Samuel 12:14-31). Interestingly David was told by Nathan that his sins were forgiven but that the child would die as part of the punishment. David must have understood Nathan's duty to confront him as God's prophet and been appreciative since he named one of his later kids Nathan! God forgives our sin when we sincerely ask Him, but the consequences can involve illness or death.

When people who don't know the Lord get a serious illness from sinful activities they may fall under conviction and then get interested in the kingdom of God. Others are puzzled or discouraged that God has "allowed" them to get sick. They

13

may conclude that God is angry with them. Sometimes that anger pushes them further from the only One Who could help them.

Some people may too quickly assume they are in this category (Specific Sins) when they are sick. They perceive God as up in heaven ready to punish them when they sin, and this punishment takes the form of sickness. This view is common in other world religions, too: if you sin, God will punish you (sometimes through sickness), and if you are righteous then He will leave you alone. Considering Job, we can see that this is not the complete, well-informed Biblical view. *Job was blameless and upright and still had terrible illness and tragedy in his life.* How should a believer understand sin-related illness?

Some sins that bring illness are related to disbelieving God when He has promised *something*, or *someone* as a leader. The men who spied out the land of Canaan but brought an evil report died of a plague (Numbers 14:37). Rebellion against anointed church leaders can bring sickness. Miriam, Moses' sister, was part of one of the rebellions mentioned earlier. Her rebellion against Moses caused her to contract temporary leprosy (Numbers 12:10). Later, when a larger group of Israelites rebelled God sent a plague. Moses bravely stood between the living and the dead, and the plague that God started was stayed (Numbers 16:46-50).

Rebellion against godly leaders is one thing, but many of Israel's leaders are recorded as being *evil*, or at least having evil behavior. Some worshiped false Gods or led their people astray. Others committed specific acts of evil. Jehoram, when he became king, strengthened himself and killed all his brothers, whom he must have considered threats to his leadership! Furthermore he built the high places (of idol worship), caused the inhabitants of Judah to commit harlotry, and led Judah astray. He was sent a letter from Elijah describing how affliction would come upon his family and how he would get an intestinal disease. This disease would cause his intestines "to come out day by day." He was sick for two years and died in severe pain. His people made no burning for him and he departed to no one's sorrow (2 Chronicles 21:19). That is, he did not even have a proper burial. How sad!

Anyone who fails to appreciate the body as the temple of God may abuse or neglect it, and they may get sick as a result. Like Peter we know that this body, this "tent," is passing away but we shouldn't hasten its passing! Lives of gluttony or disregard for exercise can lead to illness. Should these be considered specific sins? That has long been debated, so prayerfully consider your lifestyle and ask the Lord to guide you if you struggle here. The Lord gives us stewardship over our bodies, but we don't always make wise choices. The drug addict or the self-afflicter fit here. Those who cannot control alcohol use may destroy their liver or hurt themselves in car wrecks. Those who cannot control their food intake get diabetes or other obesity-related illnesses. Those who cannot control tobacco use may get lung or mouth cancer.

It is possible to be sick without having sin. One of the most instructive passages in the Bible is where the paralytic is declared *forgiven* and then Jesus says to onlookers, "Which is easier, to say your sins are forgiven or to heal miraculously?" The man was *momentarily sinless after Jesus' declaration but still paralyzed!* Then Jesus healed him physically too (Luke 5:23). What a Savior!

A person may know that his illness is due to specific sins. David said, "There is no soundness in my flesh because of Your anger, Nor is there any health in my bones because of my sin...my wounds are foul and festering because of my foolishness." (Psalm 38:3). James, the author of the New Testament book by the same name, gives advice to any who are sick, that they should call for the elders of the church to anoint them, and "if any have committed sins they will be forgiven." (James 5:15). After his healing the Bethesdan paralytic was told to "sin no more." (John 5:14). Does this mean his illness was sin-related or was this just a general exhortation by our Lord?

Namaan had enough faith to find Elisha and ask for a healing of his leprosy (and we don't know why he got it). When he was told what to do, however, he became indignant and almost missed a healing. His disobedience was countered by his servants who begged him to listen to the man of God and do what he said (2 Kings 5:1-19). How many are sick because we won't listen to and obey the man of God as he is following the Word of God? Are your friends encouraging you, like Namaan's servants, to believe God and trust His divine prescription?

3

SICK BECAUSE OF THE DEVIL & DEMONS

And they that were vexed with unclean spirits:
and they were healed.

Acts 5:16

Kevin grew up in a small town in the heartland of America. Halfway through high school, he developed daily bouts of nausea, an upset stomach, and abdominal pain. He had several medical evaluations by doctors who could not find any objective cause. He suffered so much that he almost didn't graduate. In desperation, Kevin went to the town's annual tent revival. He had heard rumors of people being healed there. He felt compelled to move down to the front at the first alter call. On the way, a strange voice came out of him that was not his own. Kevin was quickly surrounded by a group of men he did not know (mature believers). They ushered him out of the tent. Kevin was immediately thrown to the ground by an unseen force. The men encircled him and read scriptures. Kevin thrashed around on the ground while the voice came out. He stopped thrashing when the voice was gone. The men picked Kevin up and explained that he had a demon that had been cast out. Kevin was grateful, and was led to pray to God for salvation that night. From then on, Kevin did not have any more abdominal symptoms.

People in our society will say things like, "The Devil's after me!" for the most trivial of problems. He is, however, *really* after some people on this earth. The apostle Peter warned all believers that the Devil is walking about (on the earth) like a lion, seeking whom he may devour (1 Peter 5:8). The Bible contains descriptions of many people in the New Testament who are sick from either the Devil himself or his many demons, but Job's case is extremely helpful to anyone who is sick and so will be considered first.

Job: Our Example from the Old Testament

When Job exclaimed, "O that my words were written, that someone would write them down in a book" (Job 19:23) he was expressing the anguish of someone who had been bothered by the Devil and his demons. An entire book of the Bible is dedicated to this man who went through such great suffering and illness. He is not the only person mentioned in the Bible who suffered from the Devil.

Job is the earliest recorded person who suffered directly from the Devil. Through Job's story we are given insight into how the sovereignty of God plays out with a real, supernatural, fallen being who is trying to hurt us. It is interesting that the Devil had to be *allowed* by God to hurt Job, and at first he wasn't allowed to touch Job's body (Job 1:12). Job seems to be aware of this, and he attributes his trouble to God by saying, "The arrows of the Almighty are within me." (Job 6:4), and that God has "overthrown" him (Job 19:6) when responding to his friend Bildad. He says that "the hand of God hath struck me!" in 19:21. Interestingly God says that the "Devil incited Him against Job" in verse 2:3! So then the Devil is the immediate cause of Job's sickness, but God allows it and therefore is ultimately sovereign over it. In the final chapter we are told that his friends and relatives comforted and consoled him for all the adversity the Lord had brought upon him. With his sickness there is a blending into the Glory of God category (covered later) if we are willing. Things that the Devil means for bad can be turned around and used to glorify our Lord. The Devil was convinced that Job would turn his back on God in the midst of terrible suffering. The Lord was confident that Job would stay faithful through his illness and losses. Though he seemed shaky at times Job came through as gold in the end (Job 23:10). *Do we have the spiritual maturity to emerge from an illness better, stronger, and closer to God like Job?*

Job's illness is clearly attributed to the Devil (Job 2:7): "So went forth Satan from the presence of the Lord, and smote Job with sore boils from the sole of his foot unto his crown." Severe illnesses can have a spiritual cause, for the Hebrew word used for adversity in verse 2:10 can be translated "evil." Job's friends heard of his illness and came to visit him. Job's friends saw that his grief was *very great*. When they first saw him they didn't recognize him because he was so sick and they wept (Job 2:12).

In Job's story we can see how the Devil operates. It is evident that he can bring his attacks through ungodly people around us! The neighboring Sabeans and Chaldeans caused Job's servants and livestock to be killed. Even his friends *discouraged* him in their attempts to help. Were they moved by the Devil to discourage him? *We are not to put our faith in princes!* (Psalm 118:8). The Devil can, if allowed, hurt us physically. Amazingly the Devil may even have some control over the weather! He appears to have used something like a tornado to kill Job's children. Something like fire came down from heaven and burned up his sheep and servants (Job 1:16). The loss of his children and livelihood is not an illness *per se*, but must have contributed to his overall state of mind. One of the saddest parts of the book of Job is when Bildad accuses Job of unrighteousness, saying that his words are like a strong wind, which is what killed his kids! Sometimes well-meaning visitors can war against us when we are sick. We'd rather not have those kinds of visitors!

Sadly, the devil's attacks can affect even upright people who fear God. Job had a hard time understanding why these bad things were happening to him. We are invited in to his anguish, to learn from his pain. He seems near the breaking point several times, but vents to his friends (as bad as they are) and God. Physical trouble can do this; it can take us to the breaking point no matter how spiritual we are. Find someone to talk to, a mature believer or pastor who can give you encouragement and comfort in your illness. Talk to God as the psalmist did. Tell Him your deepest disappointments and needs. Even if you are angry tell Him everything. It is a step towards healing.

It is important to note that Job's sickness caused him to think about spiritual things. In the midst of his suffering he wondered out loud, "How can a man be just with God?" (Job 9:2). How many people get sick and never stop to ponder the brevity of life, the end of life, and the afterlife? Sickness can bring clarity and focus to our lives. It can, and should, cause us to pause and evaluate our days. Please consider why the Holy Spirit has allowed Job's story to be in the Bible. These things are written for our learning. Remember, Job wanted his words to be written down.

Examples from the New Testament

In Matthew 17:14-21 we read of a man who knelt down before Jesus and begged Him to heal his demon-possessed son. The kneeling man and his son are proof that some diseases are directly caused by demons. The demon caused epilepsy and severe suffering in the boy, even threatening his life by often throwing him into fire and water. Jesus rebuked the demon and the child was cured from that very hour. The disciples were unable to cast this one out. Even our best church leaders can fail, so let us kneel before our Lord and present our sick loved ones to Him in faith, like the boy's father did.

There was a man mentioned in the Bible (Matthew records two men) who lived in the area of the Gadarenes. He was well-known by the local people, and he had many demons. The Gadarene demoniac had demons that caused self-injury, nakedness, mental illness, extreme strength, fierceness, and sleeplessness (he was in the tombs day and night). They showed, by their declaration, that they knew who Jesus was and that they had limited time on the earth (Luke 8:26-33, Mark 5:1-20). Jesus cast the demons out of him. After the man was miraculously healed the local people asked Jesus to leave. Not everyone appreciates Jesus' intervention! As discussed in Chapter 7, our country's leaders have asked God to leave but we still expect God's blessings! The Word of God and prayer are both shunned in our schools and public places and we wonder why we see Him do no great things in our country (Matthew13:58).

A dumb spirit that caused tearing, gnashing, foaming, and pining away is mentioned in Mark 9:18. Jesus called it a dumb *and* deaf spirit. It is interesting that the spirit could hear, but not the child. Also, when the spirit came out it caused the child to be *almost dead*. Sometimes illness can cause us to be silent (dumb) about the things of the Lord, or not hear what He is saying anymore. It can also cause us to become so discouraged we gnash at God. Some people, even when recovered from significant illness, never return to serving the Lord. Their faith is shaken and fades. Others come through stronger. What makes the difference?

God can use your illness for His glory if you are willing. Who can you talk with (in empathy) because of your illness? Do you have the maturity to see sickness under the sovereignty of God? While you are trying to figure it out, find ways to bring God glory with your sickness! Deep and abiding trust in a time of illness is a good way to share your faith with others.

All that had diseases were brought to Jesus, and He healed them all (recorded by Luke in 4:40). Devils came out of many.

Why should the people around Jerusalem have an extra measure of demon-caused illnesses compared to us? We probably have just as many today in our cities (and in our churches) suffering this way. Even if your denominational or church background doesn't acknowledge this as a cause today, please consider that the timeless Word of God describes it as a real cause for illness. Why suffer needlessly if you can be divinely healed?

Paul's thorn in the flesh was called a messenger of Satan (2 Corinthians 12:7). He had some physical problem that served as a reminder from Satan that he (Satan) has power on this earth. Maybe it was also motivation for Paul to keep serving the Lord with zeal. He asked the Lord to heal him but was told that His grace was sufficient, that His strength was going to be made perfect in his weakness. Would you take a thorn to see God's strength perfected in you?

For some reason the Devil is allowed to cause people great suffering during this time on the earth. Since events in the garden the serpent has tried to bruise our Lord's heel and has lashed out at the image of God in us (Genesis 3:15).

SICK BECAUSE OF THE DEVIL AND DEMONS

4

SICK BECAUSE OF CHURCH DISCIPLINE

For this reason many are weak and sick among you, and many sleep.

1 Corinthians 11:30

Jim was a member of a church we once attended who became angry with the pastor for some reason. He publicly announced he would lead a group to vote the pastor out of his church on the next Sunday. Sunday morning came, but James wasn't there. He had been taken to the hospital with chest pains.

Nothing can separate us from the love of God. That is very comforting. The same God of inseparable love brings correction to His children if we stray. That too is comforting, if we can accept it. He lays His hand on us for gentle chastisement first. As (I believe) was done with Jim, there can be harsher measures – done in love – if we keep going our own way.

Church membership is a serious privilege (or it ought to be). All born-again believers are a part of the historic church of the redeemed. Local church membership has its rights and responsibilities, too. If believers go astray and bring shame to the name of Christ then there will be chastisement, just as Israel experienced.

Some departures from the honorable, abundant, and glorious life are sexual. Those who depart this way risk becoming ill outright (see Chapter 2). What happens to believers who fall into sexual sin? The fifth chapter of Corinthians contains Paul's comments to a church where it was reported that there was sexual immorality. Paul suggests "delivering" a man unto Satan who is having an affair with his father's wife. Although the implication is that the man is not saved, the advice was given to believers, to the *church* (that is us!),. Here we see Satan as the agent of bodily harm (he is always eager to help) similar to the way he operated in the book of Job. With the power of the Holy Spirit present, this form of church discipline can result in the saving of the soul. Paul says to flee fornication (sexual relations before marriage) because it causes people to "sin against their own body." (1 Corinthians 6:18). These physical actions have spiritual consequences.

King David felt God's correction after his sin with Bathsheba. We can sense David's conviction, his pain, his deep guilt in Psalm 51 and other places because he so openly wrote down his feelings. By tradition, Psalm 51 is his response to Nathan revealing his sexual sin with Bathsheba. In it he begs, "Make me hear joy and gladness, that the bones which You have broken may rejoice." In Psalm 6, David says that he makes his bed "swim all night." This may refer to when he was being chased by his enemies. David describes sin as taking his health away, and cries out to the Lord again in Psalm 38. He attributes several physical ailments to sin in that Psalm, yet appeals to God as his hope and answer. David acknowledges his sin and asks for help from the Lord, as we should. The One that brings conviction does so to get our attention. God pursues us, driven by love, and says, "You are the man." (2 Samuel 12:7). Or maybe He is quietly asking, "Where are you?" (Genesis 3:9).

Not only can individual followers of Christ err, but whole churches can, too. The church, the bride of Christ, is a special treasure of God. The Lord Himself builds her, and the gates of Hades cannot withstand her (Matthew 16:18). The local church is proof that the Word of God is being fulfilled. There are instructions in the Word about how the church is formed and what it is supposed to be doing now. Churches are so important that our Lord brings correction to churches that stray. Jesus Himself gives advice to the church at Thyatira in the book of Revelation (chapter 2). He promises to cast Jezebel onto a sickbed because of her sexual immorality and the false teaching that she encourages at that church. If she is not an actual person she certainly represents those who infiltrate the church with false teaching and sexual immorality. If you are in a church like this get out now and find a Christ-honoring church with some life!

The ordinances of the church (baptism and the Lord's Supper) should be taken in a serious, heart-felt way. Did you know that those who take the Lord's Supper in an unworthy manner are subject to sickness and death? Paul said that many in the

Corinthian church were taking the Lord's supper in an unworthy manner and were therefore eating and drinking judgment upon themselves, and were sick and dying (1 Corinthians 11:29). How many people in our churches are doing this now?

We are encouraged to support and help our local church leaders. That should be a given, but sometimes members of congregations attack or challenge their church leaders or murmur against them. Miriam and Aaron challenged Moses and it brought physical trouble on Miriam (Numbers 12). There are proper ways to speak with church leaders that are given in the New Testament. The very leader Miriam attacked was the one who had to pray for her to be healed. Plus she had seven days outside the camp to think about it even after the healing. How humbling!

God has another special treasure: Israel. The Old Testament is a love story of a supernatural Being with a people, that extends over time. It is full of accounts of Israel waxing and waning in her love for the Lord, though. God tries to woo Israel by first calling out to her, but later, uses harsher methods. Early on God tells the Israelites that He has put diseases on the Egyptians that He promises not to put on the Israelites if they will just obey Him (Exodus 15:26, Deuteronomy 7:15). Sadly, by the time of Jeremiah words like "correction" and phrases like "refusing to return" are used. In Ezekiel it seems as if all patience is exhausted and God strikes a third of Israel with "consumption, pestilence and blood." (Such national or corporate punishments are the subject of Chapter 7). In one more example from the Old Testament, God showed Moses the promise of the land He had given the Israelites. He led them out of Egypt in a great deliverance. Some of those who were sent to spy out the Promised Land brought back an evil report. They were sickened and killed by plague. Ten of the twelve spies died from unbelief (Numbers 14:37). What if this were applied today to our churches? How many would perish not believing the great promises of God?

Sometimes the Lord asks, encourages, or suggests that we do something. If we don't respond, He sometimes uses punishment to keep boundaries or to bring us back to the fold. He corrects us because He loves us, just as a father loves the son in whom He delights (Proverbs 4:12). Holy Spirit, "search our hearts, try us and know our thoughts, and see if there is any wicked way in us." (Ps 139). Help us to be the spotless Bride of Christ that He deserves! (Ephesians 5:27).

5

SICK TO ENTER THE KINGDOM

So all who dwelt at Lydda and Sharon saw [Aeneas] and turned to the Lord.

Acts 9:35

The first time I saw Rick in the hospital he was already very sick from a rapidly progressing cancer. He was a successful businessman in town, fairly well off financially with lots of hobbies and a couple of deep sea fishing boats. A concerned friend had asked if I would visit him in hopes of sharing the gospel. Those visits can be tense, but he seemed eager to see me. I was able to share the gospel using Paul's sermon on Mars Hill. Rick said he wasn't ready but wanted to hear more. I returned a few days later. His health had deteriorated. His brother, a believer, was at his bedside and had been talking with him. I hadn't been in the room long when he said, "Things are not looking good for me. I don't care about any of the things I own anymore…I'm ready to believe in the Lord and put my trust in Him." His brother and I listened as he prayed a saving prayer to the Lord, his voice choking up as he prayed. As I left, I thought of him lying there stripped of everything, including his health, but possessing the greatest gift ever given. I carried out his funeral not long after that.

Sometimes people are allowed to be sick to get them into the kingdom of God. Jesus said that "it is more profitable for one of our members (a body part) to perish than for the whole body to be cast into hell." (Matthew 5:29-30). He is emphasizing the priority of getting into the kingdom of Heaven over anything else. Thankfully, some people do gain discernment when they become seriously ill and begin to contemplate spiritual questions. *Am I ready to meet God? Is there anything I need to get right before God or man? I now see my own mortality, am I prepared for death?*

Paul had heard that there was in the Corinthian church a man who was deeply involved in a sexual sin. He ordered that the man be turned over to Satan for the "destruction of the flesh" so that his soul would be saved (1 Corinthians 5:5). He must have expected the man's awareness of impending death to motivate him to get right with God. *Let's not wait for our bodies to be destroyed before we turn to God!* That's an unfortunate way to live, and there is little opportunity to serve Him before death in many cases.

One of the earliest recorded accounts of an injury leading to spiritual insight, if not salvation, was Jacob's interaction with the Lord at Peniel (Genesis 32:24-30). Jacob struggled with a Man, got an injury, and then realized – maybe *because* of the injury – that it was God he was wrestling with. He called the place Peniel, the Face of God. He received a new name,

Israel, Prince of God, for persevering. *Do you have the ma-turity to see God's face when you have received an injury from Him?*

One person's illness can also affect those around him evangelistically. There are occasions in the New Testament where someone's miraculous healing causes other people to believe. The healing of the nobleman's son (John 4:46-54) caused many people to believe. It is called the *second miracle* and was done near the place where the *first miracle* was done, Cana of Galilee. We are told the nobleman's son was near death. He had several servants and was a man of some means. He had probably sought the finest care money could buy, with no success. Because of his faith, Jesus healed his son from afar, without even seeing him! The first miracle (turning water to wine) showed that Jesus is God, with power, and that life can get better and better for the believer towards the end ("You have kept the good wine until now.") The second mir-acle showed that even when it seems like the end has arrived, life can have a new beginning if He wills it. Jesus can heal from heaven's distance! Jesus says at Cana that unless people see signs and wonders they won't believe. Maybe your illness or healing can trigger belief in someone else. It has happened before.

We should be happy if we can influence even one person into believing in the Lord. There were several healing events that had an even greater impact than one person, causing *many* to believe. The healing of Aeneas is said to have caused the *whole population of Lydda and Sharon* to turn to the Lord (Acts 9:32-35)! He was bed-ridden for 8 years, paralyzed. When Peter came through the area visiting believers he found

Aeneas. Peter passed the message that Jesus Christ wanted to heal him. He was healed instantly and told to arise and make his bed, which he did. Imagine what was going through his mind when he was making his bed, maybe tearfully, after lying on it for 8 years! Beds are made tidy and put away by people who aren't going to be using them during the daytime. If you are a believer, befriend someone that needs healing and tell them of the Great Healer. Will He find you among the saints?

Similarly, the healing of Dorcas was said to have caused many to believe in the Lord (Acts 9:36-42). She was a woman who was "full of good works and charitable deeds." She is further proof that even godly sometimes people fall sick (see Chapter 1). Again, the believers sent for Peter, and he came to where she lay dead. Peter knelt and prayed and spoke to her body, "Arise." She sat up, then was assisted to stand up by Peter. He presented her to the believers there. Word traveled and many believed. May the Lord help us to be like Aeneas and Dorcas and bring many into the kingdom through our illness.

We've seen that illnesses can help lead people into the Kingdom of God. They can also cause us to become more serious about spiritual things. Job's illness caused him to think more deeply about spiritual things. Besides thinking about why he was sick, he wondered about the most important question in life: "How can a man be righteous before God?" (Job 9:2). It caused much self-reflection and sparked spiritual discussions even among those around him. Saul's three-day blindness after his conversion undoubtedly spurred his interest in the things of God (Acts 9). They had to lead him by the hand and he refused to eat or drink anything. He was ministered to by Ananias, humbled, and re-directed to serve the Lord. Sometimes we need to be struck blind to stop, redirect, and focus on the Lord.

Dear reader, if you are sick and are not in the kingdom of God, never having trusted Jesus with your soul, stop everything and do that now! He is available, listening right now. It truly is better for your whole body to perish and you gain a relationship with the Lord than to live a day longer without Him. If you are a believer and are ill maybe God can be glorified through your sickness as He was through Aeneas and Dorcas. Maybe many will come into the kingdom by watching you. Jacob knew he was dying, and he took the opportunity to speak great spiritual blessings to those around him (Genesis 48 and 49). He spoke to his son Joseph and his grandsons, Ephraim and Manasseh. He blessed his remaining sons and then died. Let us not leave anything unsaid at our death! Illness can be used to draw us (or others) into the kingdom if we are listening to God. If you have been declared terminally ill, why not ask, "Is this Your invitation for me to come home, Lord, and can I bring someone with me?"

6

SICK TO FULFILL PROPHECIES OR CURSES

*Son of man, I have broken the arm of Pharaoh,
king of Egypt...*

Ezekiel 30:21

Sometimes people become sick as a fulfillment of prophecies or curses. Some bring it on themselves while others are caught up in larger events. Some of the prophecies and curses in the Bible relate to the nation of Israel, the city of Jerusalem, or other cities filled with sin. Some prophecies of illness are yet to be fulfilled in the end times. It's encouraging to know that the healings Jesus performed were also the fulfillment of prophecy.

There were a couple of leaders mentioned in the Bible who were ungodly and were cursed with illness. Jehoran was such a wicked king that he was told by Elijah that he would get a great disease of the bowels "until they came out day by day." (2 Chronicles 21:15-20). As mentioned earlier (Chapter 2), that prophecy was fulfilled over a two-year period, and he died in severe pain. His was such a horrendous death that no one wanted to bury him properly. The people held no burning (burial service) for him. They buried him in the City of David, but not in the tombs of the kings as he should have been. Our funerals should be a celebration of eternal life and redemption, not a sad event. I have attended both kinds.

The death (if not the sickness) of Jeroboam's son is a sad completion of prophecy (1 Kings 14:1-31). After his son became sick he sent his wife to the prophet Ahijah. He told her that Jeroboam was such a wicked ruler that all the males of his house would die, including his ill son. It was timed so that when she came back into the city the child died. These leaders of Israel were expected to be godly people who behaved honorably. Many did not and became ill.

There were times when the Lord punished the whole nation of Israel because of idol worship or unfaithfulness. When God warned the nation about the coming captivity in Babylon there was a group that planned to avoid the judgment by escaping to Egypt. God spoke through the prophet Jeremiah and warned them that they would die by sword, famine, and *pestilence* if they went to Egypt. They went anyway, disregarding the Word of the Lord.

Ezekiel was told, before it happened, that God would break the arm of Pharaoh and give the Jewish nation relief from their oppression (Ezekiel 30:21). This released Israel from divine punishment by Egypt. Illness, injury, and death have occurred (and will occur!) to nations that mistreat Israel.

A couple of end-times prophecies involve plagues or illnesses of some sort. Zechariah is told that those who have fought against Jerusalem will be smitten with a plague that causes their flesh to consume away "while they stand on their feet (Zechariah 14:12-15)." This plague affects all animals, too. This must be supernatural, as there are not any known disease agents that can do this. These people have chosen to fight against the Lord's favorite city and they will, sadly, fulfill prophecy.

Daniel was given an end-times vision of a ram and then a male goat that would come to power and oppose the people of God, the city of God, the sanctuary of God, and then God Himself. Just the knowledge of the impending prophecy caused Daniel to be sick for days (Daniel 8:27). So his sickness was related to coming prophetic events. He was physically sick with the weight of prophecy that would occur thousands of years later!

Some are *not sick* to fulfill prophecies! The Israelites were told during the conquest of the land that they would have sickness removed from the midst of them if they were faithful to serve the Lord (Exodus 23:25).

Besides those individuals recorded in the Bible, anyone who was (or is today) divinely healed has fulfilled the Isaiah 53 prophecies mentioned in Matthew 8:17 and 1 Peter 2:24. The healings Jesus performed not only fulfilled prophecy but also validated Him as God's son. Is it legitimate to say those individuals were sick just to fulfill prophecy? Certainly their healings fulfilled prophecy.

7

SICK BECAUSE OF NATIONAL OR CORPORATE SIN

Why should you be stricken again? You will re-
volt more and more. The whole head is sick, and
the whole heart faints.

Isaiah 1:5

Blessed is the nation whose God is the Lord.
Psalm 33:12

It is impossible to think about this category without men-
tioning the special relationship God has with Israel. God
chose to break into human history in several ways: the creation of Adam and Eve, the covenants with the patriarchs, the
formation of the nation of Israel (with its special places like
Jerusalem), the written Word of God, and the incarnation of
Jesus Christ. It is extraordinary that God entered the world He
created in the first place. Sadly, His garden walks gave way to

a longer-distance relationship. At some point He chose to birth a nation, work through Abraham, Isaac, and then Jacob (whose name was changed to Israel). Promises were made that were to be fulfilled. Many times in the Word Israel is reminded that it (the country) was the apple of His eye. The people of God today (the church) should learn from Israel's special treatment and their special responsibility.

From the beginning, God promised positive and negative consequences (blessings and curses) to Israel. In book of Exodus, the people of Israel was told that if they obeyed the statutes of God the nation would be blessed. Further, God promised Israel would not experience any of the diseases in the nations around it. God would, in fact, take their diseases away. Even today, if a nation attacks or hurts Israel, then it receives God's judgment! Think of Egypt. After years of laboring there as slaves, the Israelites were released to move back to the land promised by God earlier. A series of terrible miracles was brought on the Egyptians to get them to let His people go. God said He broke the arm of pharaoh. On occasion, God punished Israel and other nations not only with sickness, but with famine or the sword or even wild beasts (mentioned in Ezekiel).

Our loving God has used sickness and other disasters as attention-grabbers to prod people to return to Him. Jeremiah lamented that even though God had stricken them (Israel) they hadn't returned and wouldn't return (Jeremiah 5:3). We've all known people who seem to move further away from God when trouble comes. Maybe we have done this, too. The very One we need to draw close to ("for I am the One that heals you!" -Exodus 15:26) is the One we shun. The One Who can help is the last One we turn to sometimes. If people think God is angry with them, it is hard for them to approach Him for help or healing. Run to Him and make peace.

At times in its history, Israel also incurred what may be called God's judgment because of continued bad behavior. That is, the whole nation fell under judgment. The Babylonian captivity is the best example, although that doesn't directly involve sickness. An occurrence of sickness as God's judgment is when the Lord became angry with Israel and led David to number the troops. Even Joab warned David that it was not a good idea. From 2 Samuel 24 it appears the Lord was ultimately behind the numbering, but in 1 Chronicles 21:1 it shows that Satan was the *agent*. This is difficult to understand, but when King David does number the troops, it results in God's chastisement. David is given a choice of punishment. He decides on a plague that runs through the nation for some time. It stops over the threshing floor of Araunah in Jerusalem. This later becomes the site of the Temple.

In Hosea 7:5, Israel's king (who was never supposed to be there anyway) had fallen into sinful influence and was said to be sick with wine, leading to ungodly leadership. Is this a physical illness or "sick" leadership? We will never know. He was influenced by his advising princes, though, in the wrong way.

In Zechariah 14:12-15, we see a principle found in scripture: even though God may discipline Israel, no other nation is allowed to hurt or attack Israel on its own! This passage from Zechariah may be about the end times, but it is still instructive. Plague was the agent that He used to punish surrounding nations that meant Israel harm.

43

The Philistines were punished with sickness for disrespecting God. In 1 Samuel 5:6-12, the Philistines had captured the ark of God. They realized, however, that He had struck them with tumors (in their private areas). They tried just sending the ark to another of their cities, but they received the same trouble. This showed a denial of the reality of the primary problem. It is interesting that the "unbelieving" Philistine priests and diviners knew about the great acts of God in history, such as how He delivered Israel out of Egypt. This warring people became sick because they took the special treasure of God, a treasure which, at that time, represented the presence of God. This was a treasure they did not appreciate or handle worthily. Is it possible that some people are ill and in denial as to why?

When Israel was delivered out of bondage from the Egyptians it was through terrible signs and wonders. From the Psalms we are told that He gave their life over to the plague and destroyed all the firstborn in Egypt (Psalm 78, 105, 135). This was a very harsh national judgment on a harsh nation.

Our nation is denying God now. It may be that some of our illnesses are due to this falling away.

8

SICK FOR THE GLORY OF GOD

When Jesus heard that, he said, "This sickness is not unto death, but for the glory of God, that the Son of God might be glorified through it."

John 11:4

The miracles of healing that fit in this category are some of the most difficult to understand in all of scripture. On the one hand, *any* healing that the Lord did (or does today) glorifies Him and causes people to see His deity. Appreciating His deity and Godhead helps people who are watching enter the kingdom of God (see Chapter 5) and makes people grateful who have experienced the healing miracle. These are all positive things that can occur in or around someone who knows they are sick for the glory of God.

The thought that someone is sick for the glory of God can be difficult to accept, however. A person's reaction may depend on their maturity level and their relationship with God. These two qualities are built on time spent with our Lord and time spent in His Word. Knowing Him well allows us to accept when He says, "My grace is sufficient," as He said to Paul when he wasn't healed (2 Corinthians 12:9). You may be very sick and in great pain, but try to let the joy that resides in you as a believer break through your difficulties.

The healing of a blind man gives some insight about how God chooses to reveal His glory through people. Before the blind man described in John 9 was healed, Jesus' disciples thought he was blind because he was a sinner (or his parents were!). They seemed to think he had his just due because of specific sins (its own category). Jesus said *neither* he nor his parents had caused his blindness but *that the works of God should be revealed in him* (John 9:3). In this healing there is, of course, also a nice validation of the prophet or man of God. More importantly, it is proof that there is a God Who cares for us and is able to heal supernaturally! Sadly, the Jews, and specifically the Pharisees, did not give God glory after seeing this miracle and promptly cast him out (of the synagogue?). Jesus, however, found the man and asked if he believed in the Son of God. He did and worshipped Him. *What a great outcome when sickness leads to healing and then healing to the Son of God!* Both believers and non-believers can experience this. Non-believers can be led all the way to the Lord through illness and then into the kingdom of God. Believers can get a deeper walk with the Lord after an illness, if they are willing.

Perhaps the best example, the most specific answer in the New Testament of why someone was sick, is found in Lazarus' story (John 11). We are told that Lazarus was sick "for the glory of God," specifically, "that the Son of God may be glorified through it." This account is worth examining in more detail. Mary and Martha sent word to Jesus saying that *the one He loved was sick.* They meant Lazarus, their brother. The Greek word translated "love" here means the one you "like." The Bible records though, just two verses later, that Jesus indeed "loved" Martha, Mary, and Lazarus, but the word used there is *agape*, the undeserved, divine, chosen love. The miracle He then did shows His victory over death and the grave for any believer. *Resurrection is the ultimate healing!* Jesus Himself is the first fruits of the resurrection, but Lazarus is a token of God's ultimate healing for all of us. Eventually your grave-clothes are coming off!

Physical healing, Jesus forgiving us of our sins, and the resurrection all glorify God and give man hope and encouragement. God is the only One Who can glorify Himself sinlessly, without pride. Healing miracles praise and glorify Him Who rightfully deserves worship. Do you have the maturity to ask *How can God be glorified through my illness?* Can you help a friend or loved one who is sick ask this question? We have encouragement from Paul, who looked at his chains and the things that had happened to him as something that furthered the gospel. To the end, his wish was that "Christ will be magnified in my body, whether by life or by death." (Philippians 1:20)

9

SELF-INVENTORY

*Search me, O God, and know my heart; Try me
and know my anxieties; And see if there is any
wicked way in me, And lead me in the way ever-
lasting.*

Psalm 139:23-24

Being sick is depressing and heartbreaking both to you and
those around you. If it were possible to know *why* and to
do something about it then, wouldn't you want to? That was
the first hope I had when writing this book, that people might
be able to understand why they were ill. Understanding should
lead to comfort and possibly change and hope. Read this chapter and prayerfully see if the Lord gives you insight and understanding.

The first thing to do is ask the Lord to reveal to you why
you are sick. Try to discern if He is allowing this illness to get
you into the kingdom of God. If that is the case then respond
to His action NOW! He is extending His grace to you to get
you interested in spiritual things and lead you into salvation.

For it is better to enter the kingdom with one eye than not enter at all. Humbly ask the Holy Spirit to show you if you are in this category. Maybe you have a loved one who is sick. Some people have to receive a severe illness to get their attention off things of this world and onto the Savior. It is sad to see a loved one go through this. Your heart will first break for them but later rejoice that they have found redemption. Be available for help and guidance.

If you are sick just because Sin has entered the world and affects all people equally then seek medical help. Our Lord sanctioned medical professions when He said, "It is not the well people that need a physician but the sick (Luke 5:31)." Remember, even the most spiritual among us still get sick! Luke was a physician and a valued disciple, writing one of the gospels and accompanying Paul on missionary trips. Sometimes our medical personnel extend God's grace and don't even know it!

Throw yourself into the Word of God. Besides providing comfort it may give you truth you need to hear. There are things God has *already* revealed in His Word, especially those that concern specific sins. If you have become sick through specific sins you can discern that pretty quickly. Just ask the Lord if He will reveal this to you through His Word.

How does a person know if he has a demon or if the Devil is hurting him? All I can say is that some people seem to know. In the Bible other people could see it and would bring the possessed person to the Lord for healing. Have people around you ever suggested this? Some of these *come out by prayer and fasting only.* Find mature believers to ask who can help you discern if this is happening to you. They may also be able to help with treatment.

If you think you might be ill because of church discipline humble yourself and ask the Holy Spirit to show you. Have you been challenging your church's leadership in an ungodly way? Remember Miriam, Korah, and others from the Bible. While Israel isn't the church, it does seem reasonable that we not do the same things that got them in trouble! Our Lord is always ready to forgive. Be glad we are in a time of grace. The ground could have opened and swallowed you! Remember, Paul said some in the church were sick because they were taking the Lord's Supper in an unworthy manner. Take time to ask for forgiveness, recommit yourself, and humble yourself before taking the Lord's Supper again.

How do you know if you are in the Glory of God category? After you have prayerfully thought through the other categories and not recognized yourself then you may be in this category. One of the most important principles of the kingdom of God is that any of the categories can be turned into the Glory of God. This, of course, takes maturity and trust.

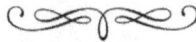

⌘

Our family gathered around Dad's hospital bed about the same time for three days in a row for prayer. Believing it was the greatest thing we could do, we placed a hand-written sign on his door reading: "Do Not Disturb! Family Prayer Time." With a small amount of anointing oil, we asked the Lord to heal him outright. We also asked God to comfort him from the unrelenting nausea, and to give the doctors and staff of the hospital wisdom. We agreed to pray together for three days in a row because Paul had three times asked the Lord to heal him. We would not have been at all surprised by a divine healing, but trusted that His grace was sufficient if we didn't get that. We, of course, kept praying individually, but felt it important to have group prayer those three days. We also knew it would be difficult to get our family together like that again for some time. We had high hopes, but Dad's condition worsened over the next couple of weeks.

10

HELP

As mentioned previously, when Job exclaimed, "O that my words were written, that someone would write them down in a book," he was begging for someone to hear him. Counselors know that there is something beneficial about venting, about sharing our deepest disappointments and ailments with others. Of course, it is most helpful to share with the One most able to affect our body (and mind!). The Psalmist had the right idea when he said, "Have mercy on me, o Lord, for I am weak; O Lord heal me, for my bones are troubled (Psalm 6:2)." God, after all, is described as the "One Who heals all your diseases (Psalm 103:3)." The One who made us has the ability to heal us supernaturally. Sometimes He does. We know that He did during His earthly ministry, and we can learn from it. Do not be "destroyed for lack of knowledge (Hosea 4:6)."

The disciples understood that God alone has the power to heal supernaturally. Peter reminded amazed crowds that it wasn't his godliness that worked healing but the power of God (Acts 3). By faith saints throughout history have obediently anointed the sick with oil, praying for them and asking the

Lord Himself to heal. Isaiah prophesied about Jesus saying that He would "take our infirmities and bare our sicknesses." (Isaiah 53:4). It is interesting to note that even Judas was given by our Lord the power to heal (Matthew 10:4).

Of course Jesus Himself healed people directly when He was present on the earth. So many people came to be healed that He, at times, fled to the other shore of the lake or into the wilderness. At times, He asked those healed not to say anything, possibly because it would delay or distract His Messianic mission. We should still ask, today, for miraculous healing. It seems to anger our Lord when we have unbelief in this area. He put the crowd outside when they laughed Him to scorn just before healing the ruler's daughter (Matthew 9:25). Sometimes it feels as if our whole country has been "put outside" because of our unbelief!

Our Lord loves us with *agape* love (remember Lazarus) and cares that we are suffering. Otherwise, why does Jesus *cry* if He knows He is going to raise Lazarus from the dead? The sickness and death of Lazarus with the anguish of family members affected our Lord to tears. Sometimes it may seem as if Jesus is staying away two days when we are sick, as He did for Lazarus. That kind of frustration is difficult and causes saints to cry, "How long, Lord?" The writer of Psalm 102:10 felt abandoned by God but still kept a proper view. Even the cries of babies praise God and silence the enemy and avenger (Psalm 8:2). Cry out to God and ask Him to comfort you under the shadow of His wings (Psalm 17:8, 36:7, 44:19, 57:1, 61:4, 63:7, 91:4).

Besides crying out to God it may be helpful to share with trusted friends. Job's friends are sometimes criticized for their bad advice. Maybe they deserve credit, though, for seeking him out, just sitting with him for a week, and not saying anything (just listening and being with him!). In the best cases iron can sharpen iron and we can be cheered up (literally have our face keened). It is part of bearing one another's burdens.

Dear reader, please take the Inventory in the previous chapter to help you discern if you are in an obvious, known category. It was my hope from the beginning that this book would help ill people understand why they were sick and be comforted. Whatever category you find yourself in, take time to cry out to the Lord, the God of heaven and earth.

If we are sinning specific sins then we need to STOP, and, as James suggests, call for the elders of the church to anoint and pray over us.

We can trust in the Lord for the ultimate protection against the "pestilence that walks in darkness" (Psalm 91). When your soul is bowed down to the dust and your body clings to the ground ask the Lord to arise and redeem you!

The spirit of a man will sustain him in sickness (Proverbs 18:14)!

We do indeed look forward to the day He makes all things new (Revelation 21:5)!

Epilogue

Dad nearly died in the hospital the week after his cancer was discovered. The prolonged unwilling fast due to vomiting had weakened him considerably, and the surgery didn't help. His kidneys shut down and my brother, who is a physician, noticed what was happening and acted quickly to save him – the first of several times. His type and stage of cancer had a terrible prognosis (I checked the latest information but never shared the bad statistics with my family, just couldn't do it). He decided to try the chemotherapy offered. It added to his trouble, and he suffered through about 8 months of unrelenting nausea, vomiting several times each day and often several times each night. When I visited I'd be awakened by the sound of him getting sick in the middle of the night. My mom was there the whole time (may the Lord reward you according to your works). Sometimes I would come downstairs and put my hand on his back and say, "Aw man, sorry...sorry Dad." Besides making sure he got his medicine on time there was little that could be done when he was getting sick.

He seemed to improve just enough to get up and around for a few great weeks and then the chemotherapy lost its effectiveness. Regular imaging studies that summer showed spread to other organs, including spine and hip. Besides the nausea, pain now radiated from these other areas. I was visiting the weekend he decided to stop all medicines. He would enter hospice care soon. I told him we kids (all grown with families of our own) were grateful for our childhood, and that he was a fantastic dad. We all broke down that afternoon as the reality sunk in.

There were some positives: the Lord granted him a few months to get his house in order. Some people are not given even this time. One of his desires was to die at home, on his farm, and not in a hospital. He was able to get back home for the last four months, helped by several people, including his brother who checked on him all the time, and his family doctor who made home visits. Toward the end he told Mom, "I'm waiting for Jesus to come and get me." The last thing I remember him saying was, "Tell everyone I love them." He passed peacefully into eternity two days after his 74th birthday in November with his family holding both of his hands.

Sin's Entrance into the world will cause your loved ones to be taken from this life. Thankfully, our Lord has shown us a way to have resurrected, eternal life and hope of reunion with our loved ones in heaven again. This is why we have the gospel message. "Thanks be to God for His indescribable gift!" (2 Corinthians 9:15).

Acknowledgments

From Davis McGuirt

I thank the Lord for the book that sits before me, based on the Book that sits before me. He changed my life during the process with His Word, and I am now sure that the book was just a small part of a larger project. Working for Him has been honorable and glorious.

The Lord gave me the idea for this book in 1999. My wife, Mary Kay, and I were serving as missionaries in a church-planting ministry. Because I was so busy then I just pondered it, and I never brought it to written form. Over the next 15 years, I used the ideas in my classes at college and continued to think about writing everything down in a book. By 2012 I began to wonder if I would ever complete the book and gave up on writing it myself. Once I became willing to receive help the Lord opened a door to me. In 2014, a student walked into my office and volunteered for a Christian Service project. I said, "Have you ever thought about helping someone write a book?" Over the next several months things happened like in the book of Acts, with believers helping each other and signs and wonders taking place. Most who helped were believers, but some weren't. Our prayer became, "Grant us the ones sailing with us."

I would like to thank many people who have helped along the way. I have been surrounded by encouragers, and I am very grateful. My wife and kids have been very supportive, and I thank God for them. Friends, especially those who have prayed for the project, were true blessings. My mother and late father encouraged me to love the Lord with my mind as well as my heart. My mother was the quickest and best editor. My brother gave the best advice on the purpose of the book (and contributed a story). He encouraged me to read the Word the first time and helped me come into the kingdom in 1992. Dr. Gary Chapman has been a great role model as a Christian and a writer. My professors and fellow laborers, particularly my Nigerian friend Mark Akinosho, helped me understand the Word and the ministry of the blessed Holy Spirit. I appreciate the support from my local church, Tree of Life Ministries.

My colleague in NY, Jim Wolfe, taught me to serve the Lord as a teacher. My students and co-workers at Liberty University have been willing test cases of these ideas about disease, and deeply encouraging. I thank the staff of the Jerry Falwell Library and Starbucks for their assistance, help, and smiling faces. I thank Bethel Music and Jonathan Helser for their music… truly a year dripping with abundance. I am grateful to all those who read the numerous drafts. To Corderius, you are a great encourager. Thanks to Joan, Bob Bowen, and Tom Nelson for your help over the years. Thanks to Bernie Geisel who innocently asked, "What's your time frame on writing the book?"

Finally, I thank Heather, who said, "I would be honored to help write a book." May the Lord reward you in this life and the life to come.

Lord, You crown the year with Your goodness…

- Davis McGuirt

ACKNOWLEDGMENTS

From Heather Geisel

Thank you Abba for EVERYTHING you have done with Your project. I have learned more about who You are and have fallen deeper in love with you. My life will never be the same, and I praise You for that. Your overwhelming love towards Your children is never-ending and always overflowing. Thank you for the cross.

Dad and Mom, how can I ever thank you enough for sharing the greatest gift a parent could ever offer their children, *Jesus*? Train up a child in the way he should go and when he is old he will not depart from it (Proverbs 22:6). Thank you for your unconditional love and endless encouragement. Thank you for being examples of godliness and perseverance. I am proud to be called your daughter. To my sister, Tami, I am so grateful for your undying support in anything and everything I do and attempt. You are my best friend and my angel. I love you girl. To my Brother-n-law, Mike, you have always had my back and I appreciate that. To my precious nieces and nephew...Kaily, Alaina, Kassi, Brenna, Allie, and Hunter...my prayer is that you grow in the grace and knowledge of who Jesus is, and may you find out how precious you truly are in His sight. Nothing else matters in this life except to know Jesus and believe He died for you to give you Salvation. Your Auntie loves you all so much. To my brother, Jeff, and his wife, Ann, you both have always encouraged me, stood up for me, and loved me. To my brother, Scott, and his wife, Colleen, thank you for all your prayers, love, and support throughout the years and for the laughs we have all shared and will continue to share. I love you guys.

A special thank you to all of my friends and family who have prayed along this journey with us... you are treasured. I am happy we have encountered one another along the way. My prayer for you all is that you feel encouraged, feel comforted, and feel deeply loved by our Heavenly Father knowing that through Salvation only, one day we will see the ones that have gone before us but reside with Jesus and are living today.

Lastly, thank you Dr. McGuirt for offering me this incredible opportunity to help you with this project. It's been a life changer and I am grateful. Thank you.

Who crowns you with lovingkindess and tender-mercies...

- Heather Geisel